IMG Friendly Dermatology Residency Programs List

With Comprehensive Match Selection Criteria and Programs Requirements

By

IMG Guide

I0476427

And

Applicant Guide

Introduction

IMG Friendly Dermatology Residency Programs

With Comprehensive Match Selection Criteria and Programs Requirements

In Collaboration between the Applicant
Guide and the IMG Guide we present to you
the most complete and up-to-date IMG
friendly dermatology residency programs
list with full match selection criteria and
requirements for these programs. This book
is essentially written for international

medical graduates seeking residency in the US. The idea of writing this book came from our insight that many IMGs every year don't match because they don't know where to apply. Most of the time, they end applying to programs that don't have IMGs or those that don't match their criteria hence they end losing money with no interviews earned. The information was gathered from program directors, coordinators, chiefs, faculty and residents. It includes Programs names, Programs codes, States, Addresses, Phones, Faxes, Percentage of IMGs in the programs, Minimum USMLE Step 1 and Step 2 Score Requirements, Attempts on any step, CS requirement at time of application, USCE Requirements, Cut-Off time since graduation, Programs offering couple match and Visas Sponsored or accepted.

which is/are subject to change by/at the programs at any time. Although we did our best to get the most accurate information as much as possible from the program directors, coordinators, faculty and residents, however, you understand that by reading this book you are using the information here on your own responsibility.

Alabama

University of Alabama Medical Center Dermatology Residency Program

Specialty: Dermatology
Program name: University of Alabama Medical Center Program
Program code: 080-01-21-010
Program type: University-based
State: Alabama
Address: University of Alabama Medical Center, EFH 414,

      1720 University Blvd, Birmingham, AL 35294
Phone: (205) 934-5189
Fax: (205) 934-5766
Percentage of IMGs in the program: 8%
Minimum USMLE Step 1 Score Requirement: 240
Minimum USMLE Step 2 Score Requirement: 240

Attempts on any step: Must pass first attempt
CS required at time of application: No
USCE Requirement: Yes
Cut-Off time since graduation: Fresh graduates only
Program offers couple match: No
Visas Sponsored or accepted: J1 visa and H1b visa

California

University of Southern California/LAC+USC Medical Center Dermatology Residency Program

Specialty: Dermatology
Program name: University of Southern California/LAC+USC Medical Center Program
Program code: 080-05-11-015
Program type: University-based
State: California
Address: USC Norris Cancer Hospital, Ezralow Tower #5301,
          1441 Eastlake Ave, Los Angeles, CA 90033
Phone: (323) 442-0084
Fax: (323) 442-0067
Percentage of IMGs in the program: 10%

Minimum USMLE Step 1 Score Requirement:
No limits set
Minimum USMLE Step 2 Score Requirement:
No limits set
Attempts on any step: No limits set
CS required at time of application: No but
PTAL/Status letter required
USCE Requirement: None
Cut-Off time since graduation: No limits set
Program offers couple match: Yes
Visas Sponsored or accepted: J1 visa and H1b
visa

Jackson Memorial Hospital/Jackson Health System Dermatology Residency Program

Specialty: Dermatology
Program name: Jackson Memorial
Hospital/Jackson Health System Program
Program code: 080-11-21-026
State: Florida
Address: University of Miami/Jackson Memorial
Hospital, Dermatology Program (R-250),
          PO Box 016250, Miami, FL 33101
Phone: (305) 243-6742
Fax: (305) 243-6191
Percentage of IMGs in the program: 10%
Minimum USMLE Step 1 Score Requirement:
220

Minimum USMLE Step 2 Score Requirement:
220
Attempts on any step: No limits set
CS required at time of application: Yes
including ECFMG certificate
USCE Requirement: Yes
Cut-Off time since graduation: No limits set
Program offers couple match: Yes
Visas Sponsored or accepted: J1 visa

University of Florida Dermatology Residency Program

Specialty: Dermatology
Program name: University of Florida Program
Program code: 080-11-21-115
Program type: University-based
State: Florida
Address: University of Florida College of
Medicine, PO Box 100279,
          4037 NW 86 TR, Gainesville, FL 32610-
0279
Phone: (352) 594-1925
Fax: (352) 594-1926
Percentage of IMGs in the program: 15%
Minimum USMLE Step 1 Score Requirement:
240
Minimum USMLE Step 2 Score Requirement:
240

Attempts on any step: Must pass on first attempt
CS required at time of application: Yes including ECFMG certificate
USCE Requirement: Yes
Cut-Off time since graduation: 3 years
Program offers couple match: Yes
Visas Sponsored or accepted: J1 visa

Georgia

Emory University Dermatology Residency Program

Specialty: Dermatology
Program name: Emory University Program
Program code: 080-12-21-028
NRMP Code: 1113080A0
Program type: University-based
State: Georgia
Address: Emory University School of Medicine, Department of Dermatology 1st Fl,
          1525 Clifton Rd, Atlanta, GA 30322
Phone: (404) 727-3669
Fax: (404) 727-5874
Percentage of IMGs in the program: 10%

Minimum USMLE Step 1 Score Requirement:
No limits set
Minimum USMLE Step 2 Score Requirement:
No limits set
Attempts on any step: No limits set
CS required at time of application: Yes
including ECFMG exam
USCE Requirement: Yes
Cut-Off time since graduation: No limits set
Program offers couple match: Yes
Visas Sponsored or accepted: J1 visa and H1b
visa

Illinois

Loyola University Dermatology Residency Program

Specialty: Dermatology
Program name: Loyola University Program
Program code: 080-16-12-135
NRMP Code: 1170080A0
Program type: University-based
State: Illinois
Address: Loyola University Medical Center,
Building 54 Room 136,
        2160 S First Ave, Maywood, IL 60153
Phone: (708) 216-4807

Fax: (708) 216-2444
Percentage of IMGs in the program: 20%
Minimum USMLE Step 1 Score Requirement: 230
Minimum USMLE Step 2 Score Requirement: 230
Attempts on any step: Must pass on first attempt including CS exam
CS required at time of application: Yes including ECFMG certificate
USCE Requirement: None
Cut-Off time since graduation: 4 years
Program offers couple match: Yes
Visas Sponsored or accepted: J1 visa

John H Stroger Hospital of Cook County Dermatology Residency Program

Specialty: Dermatology
Program name: John H Stroger Hospital of Cook County Program
Program code: 080-16-12-030
State: Illinois
Address: Stroger Hospital of Cook County, Administration Building Room 519,
        1900 W Polk St, Chicago, IL 60612-9985
Phone: (312) 864-4478

Fax: (312) 864-9663
Percentage of IMGs in the program: 10%
Minimum USMLE Step 1 Score Requirement: 230
Minimum USMLE Step 2 Score Requirement: 230
Attempts on any step: No limits set
CS required at time of application: No
USCE Requirement: Yes
Cut-Off time since graduation: No limits set
Program offers couple match: No
Visas Sponsored or accepted: J1 visa and H1b visa

Indiana

Indiana University School of Medicine Dermatology Residency Program

Specialty: Dermatology
Program name: Indiana University School of Medicine Program
Program code: 080-17-21-035
NRMP Code: 1187080C0
Program type: Community-based university affiliated hospital
State: Indiana

Address: Indiana University Medical Center, EH 139,

545 Barnhill Dr, Indianapolis, IN 46202-5267
Phone: (317) 278-6833
Fax: (317) 274-3700
Percentage of IMGs in the program: 10%
Minimum USMLE Step 1 Score Requirement: 220
Minimum USMLE Step 2 Score Requirement: 220
Attempts on any step: No limits set
CS required at time of application: Yes including ECFMG certificate
USCE Requirement: None
Cut-Off time since graduation: No limits set
Program offers couple match: Yes
Visas Sponsored or accepted: No visa

Kansas

University of Kansas School of Medicine Dermatology Residency Program

Specialty: Dermatology
Program name: University of Kansas School of Medicine Program
Program code: 080-19-11-037

Program type: University-based
State: Kansas
Address: University of Kansas Medical Center, MS2025 Rm 4010 Wescoe,
 3901 Rainbow Blvd, Kansas City, KS 66160-7319
Phone: (913) 588-3840
Fax: (913) 588-8300
Percentage of IMGs in the program: 8%
Minimum USMLE Step 1 Score Requirement: 230
Minimum USMLE Step 2 Score Requirement: 230
Attempts on any step: No limits set
CS required at time of application:
USCE Requirement: Yes including ECFMG certificate
Cut-Off time since graduation: No limits set
Program offers couple match: Yes
VIsas Sponsored or accepted: J1 visa and H1b visa

Massachusetts

Massachusetts General Hospital/Beth Israel Deaconess Medical Center/Brigham and Women's Hospital Dermatology Residency Program

Specialty: Dermatology
Program name: Massachusetts General Hospital/Beth Israel Deaconess Medical Center/Brigham and Women's Hospital Program
Program code: 080-24-31-043
State: Massachusetts
Address: Massachusetts General Hospital, Bartlett Hall 616,

      55 Fruit St, Boston, MA 02114
Phone: (617) 726-5254
Fax: (617) 726-1875
Percentage of IMGs in the program: 6%
Minimum USMLE Step 1 Score Requirement: 215
Minimum USMLE Step 2 Score Requirement: 215
Attempts on any step: No limits set
CS required at time of application: No
USCE Requirement: Yes
Cut-Off time since graduation: No limits set
Program offers couple match: No
Visas Sponsored or accepted: J1 visa and H1b visa

Tufts Medical Center Dermatology Residency Program

Specialty: Dermatology
Program name: Tufts Medical Center Program
Program code: 080-24-21-141
State: Massachusetts
Address: Tufts Medical Center, Department of Dermatology #114,
    800 Washington St, Boston, MA 02111
Phone: (617) 636-7480
Fax: (617) 636-9169
Percentage of IMGs in the program: 20%
Minimum USMLE Step 1 Score Requirement: 230
Minimum USMLE Step 2 Score Requirement: 230
Attempts on any step: Must pass on first attempt
CS required at time of application: Yes including ECFMG certificate
USCE Requirement: None
Cut-Off time since graduation: 10 years
Program offers couple match: No
Visas Sponsored or accepted: J1 visa

Boston Medical Center Dermatology Residency Program

Specialty: Dermatology
Program name: Boston Medical Center Program
Program code: 080-24-21-044
State: Massachusetts
Address: Boston University Medical Center, Department of Dermatology J-202,
          609 Albany St, Boston, MA 02118-2394
Phone: (617) 414-1366
Fax: (617) 414-1363
Percentage of IMGs in the program: 6%
Minimum USMLE Step 1 Score Requirement: No limits set
Minimum USMLE Step 2 Score Requirement: No limits set
Attempts on any step: No limits set
CS required at time of application: Yes including ECFMG Certificate
USCE Requirement: None
Cut-Off time since graduation: No limits set
Program offers couple match: No
Visas Sponsored or accepted: J1 visa

Minnesota

University of Minnesota Dermatology Residency Program

Specialty: Dermatology
Program name: University of Minnesota Program
Program code: 080-26-31-048
Program type: University-based
State: Minnesota
Address: University of Minnesota Medical Center, Department of Dermatology MMC 98, 420 Delaware St SE, Minneapolis, MN 55455-0392
Phone: (612) 624-9964
Fax: (612) 624-6678
Percentage of IMGs in the program: 5%
Minimum USMLE Step 1 Score Requirement: 230
Minimum USMLE Step 2 Score Requirement: 230
Attempts on any step: No limits set
CS required at time of application: No
USCE Requirement: None
Cut-Off time since graduation: No limits set
Program offers couple match: Yes
Visas Sponsored or accepted: J1 visa

New Hampshire

Dartmouth-Hitchcock Medical Center Dermatology Residency Program

Specialty: Dermatology
Program name: Dartmouth-Hitchcock Medical Center Program
Program code: 080-32-21-053
Program type: University-based
State: New Hampshire
Address: Dartmouth-Hitchcock Medical Center, Section of Dermatology,
        One Medical Center Dr, Lebanon, NH 03756
Phone: (603) 650-3156
Fax: (603) 650-3172
Percentage of IMGs in the program: 18%
Minimum USMLE Step 1 Score Requirement: 220
Minimum USMLE Step 2 Score Requirement: 220
Attempts on any step: No limits set
CS required at time of application: Yes
USCE Requirement: Yes
Cut-Off time since graduation: No limits set
Program offers couple match: Yes
Visas Sponsored or accepted: J1 visa

New Jersey

Rutgers Robert Wood Johnson Medical School Dermatology Residency Program

Specialty: Dermatology
Program name: Rutgers Robert Wood Johnson Medical School Program
Program code: 080-33-31-128
State: New Jersey
Address: UMDNJ-Robert Wood Johnson Medical School,
        Department of Dermatology Suite 2400,
        1 World's Fair Dr, Somerset, NJ 08873
Phone: (732) 235-7765
Fax: (732) 235-6568
Percentage of IMGs in the program: 15%
Minimum USMLE Step 1 Score Requirement: No limits set
Minimum USMLE Step 2 Score Requirement: No limits set
Attempts on any step: No limits set
CS required at time of application: Yes including ECFMG certificate
USCE Requirement: None
Cut-Off time since graduation: No limits set
Program offers couple match: No
Visas Sponsored or accepted: No visa

New York

St Luke's-Roosevelt Hospital Center Dermatology Residency Program

Specialty: Dermatology
Program name: St Luke's-Roosevelt Hospital Center Program
Program code: 080-35-21-124
NRMP Code: 2070080A0
Program type: Community-based university affiliated hospital
State: New York
Address: St Luke's-Roosevelt Hospital Center, Department of Dermatology Suite 11B,
          1090 Amsterdam Ave, New York, NY 10025
Phone: (212) 523-3812
Fax: (212) 523-3808
Percentage of IMGs in the program: 20%
Minimum USMLE Step 1 Score Requirement: No limits set
Minimum USMLE Step 2 Score Requirement: No limits set
Attempts on any step: No limits set
CS required at time of application: Yes including ECFMG certificate

USCE Requirement: None
Cut-Off time since graduation: No limits set
Program offers couple match: Yes
Visas Sponsored or accepted: J1 visa

New York University School of Medicine Dermatology Residency Program

Specialty: Dermatology
Program name: New York University School of Medicine Program
Program code: 080-35-21-064
Program type: University-based
State: New York
Address: New York University Medical Center,
        Ambulatory Care Ctr Dermatology
Pgm 11th Floor,
        240 E 38th St, New York, NY 10016
Phone: (212) 263-3722
Fax: (212) 263-8752
Percentage of IMGs in the program: 5%
Minimum USMLE Step 1 Score Requirement: No limits set
Minimum USMLE Step 2 Score Requirement: No limits set
Attempts on any step: No limits set
CS required at time of application: Yes including ECFMG certificate
USCE Requirement: None

Cut-Off time since graduation: No limits set
Program offers couple match: Yes
Visas Sponsored or accepted: J1 visa and H1b visa

New York Medical College (Metropolitan) Dermatology Residency Program

Specialty: Dermatology
Program name: New York Medical College (Metropolitan) Program
Program code: 080-35-21-063
Program type: University-based
State: New York
Address: Metropolitan Hospital Center, Department of Dermatology Room 1208,
         1901 First Ave, New York, NY 10029
Phone: (212) 423-7467
Fax: (212) 423-8464
Percentage of IMGs in the program: 25%
Minimum USMLE Step 1 Score Requirement: 225
Minimum USMLE Step 2 Score Requirement: 225
Attempts on any step: Must pass on first attempt including CS exam
CS required at time of application: Yes including ECFMG certificate

USCE Requirement: None
Cut-Off time since graduation: 3 years
Program offers couple match: No
Visas Sponsored or accepted: J1 visa and H1b visa

SUNY Health Science Center at Brooklyn Dermatology Residency Program

Specialty: Dermatology
Program name: SUNY Health Science Center at Brooklyn Program
Program code: 080-35-21-065
NRMP Code: 1426080A0
Program type: University-based
State: New York
Address: SUNY Downstate Medical Center, Department of Dermatology,
        450 Clarkson Ave, Brooklyn, NY 11203
Phone: (718) 270-1229
Fax: (718) 270-2794
Percentage of IMGs in the program: 8%
Minimum USMLE Step 1 Score Requirement: 230
Minimum USMLE Step 2 Score Requirement: 230
Attempts on any step: No limits set
CS required at time of application: Yes including ECFMG certificate

USCE Requirement: None
Cut-Off time since graduation: No limits set
Program offers couple match: No
Visas Sponsored or accepted: No visa

Albert Einstein College of Medicine Dermatology Residency Program

Specialty: Dermatology
Program name: Albert Einstein College of Medicine Program
Program code: 080-35-31-058
NRMP Code: 3153080A0
Program type: University-based
State: New York
Address: Montefiore Medical Center, Division of Dermatology,
　　　　111 E 210th St, Bronx, NY 10467-2490
Phone: (718) 920-2680
Fax: (718) 944-4219
Percentage of IMGs in the program: 8%
Minimum USMLE Step 1 Score Requirement: 215
Minimum USMLE Step 2 Score Requirement: 215
Attempts on any step: No limits set
CS required at time of application: No
USCE Requirement: Yes
Cut-Off time since graduation: No limits set
Program offers couple match: Yes

Visas Sponsored or accepted: No visa

North Carolina

University of North Carolina Hospitals Dermatology Residency Program

Specialty: Dermatology
Program name: University of North Carolina Hospitals Program
Program code: 080-36-11-066
Program type: University-based
State: North Carolina
Address: University of North Carolina Hospitals, Department of Dermatology CB#7715t Suite 400,
        410 Market St, Chapel Hill, NC 27516
Phone: (919) 843-5539
Fax: (919) 966-6460
Percentage of IMGs in the program: 5%
Minimum USMLE Step 1 Score Requirement: No limits set
Minimum USMLE Step 2 Score Requirement: No limits set
Attempts on any step: No limits set
CS required at time of application: No
USCE Requirement: None

Cut-Off time since graduation: No limits set
Program offers couple match: Yes
Visas Sponsored or accepted: J1 visa

Ohio

Cleveland Clinic Foundation Dermatology Residency Program

Specialty: Dermatology
Program name: Cleveland Clinic Foundation Program
Program code: 080-38-12-070
NRMP Code: 1968080C0
Program type: University-based
State: Ohio
Address: Cleveland Clinic, Desk A60,
            9500 Euclid Ave, Cleveland, OH 44195-5242
Phone: (216) 444-5933
Fax: (216) 636-5830
Percentage of IMGs in the program: 5%
Minimum USMLE Step 1 Score Requirement: No limits set
Minimum USMLE Step 2 Score Requirement: No limits set
Attempts on any step: No limits set
CS required at time of application: No

USCE Requirement: None
Cut-Off time since graduation: No limits set
Program offers couple match: Yes
Visas Sponsored or accepted: J1 visa and H1b visa

Pennsylvania

University of Pennsylvania Dermatology Residency Program

Specialty: Dermatology
Program name: University of Pennsylvania Program
Program code: 080-41-21-080
Program type: University-based
State: Pennsylvania
Address: Hospital of University of Pennsylvania, Department of Dermatology 2 Maloney Building,
3600 Spruce St, Philadelphia, PA 19104
Phone: (215) 662-7883
Fax: (215) 662-7884
Percentage of IMGs in the program: 5%
Minimum USMLE Step 1 Score Requirement: No limits set

Minimum USMLE Step 2 Score Requirement:
No limits set
Attempts on any step: No limits set
CS required at time of application: Yes
including ECFMG certificate
USCE Requirement: Yes
Cut-Off time since graduation: No limits set
Program offers couple match: Yes
Visas Sponsored or accepted: J1 visa and H1b
visa

Thomas Jefferson University Dermatology Residency Program

Specialty: Dermatology
Program name: Thomas Jefferson University
Program
Program code: 080-41-11-079
Program type: University-based
State: Pennsylvania
Address: Jefferson Dermatology Associates,
Suite 740,
833 Chestnut St, Philadelphia, PA
19107
Phone: (215) 955-4947
Fax: (215) 503-3333
Percentage of IMGs in the program: 8%
Minimum USMLE Step 1 Score Requirement:
No limits set

Minimum USMLE Step 2 Score Requirement: No limit set
Attempts on any step: Must pass on first attempt
CS required at time of application: Yes including ECFMG certificate
USCE Requirement: None
Cut-Off time since graduation: No limits set
Program offers couple match: No
Visas Sponsored or accepted: J1 visa and H1b visa

Rhode Island

Roger Williams Medical Center Dermatology Residency Program

Specialty: Dermatology
Program name: Roger Williams Medical Center Program
Program code: 080-43-21-083
State: Rhode Island
Address: Roger Williams Medical Center, Dermatology & Skin Surgery,
        50 Maude St, Providence, RI 02908
Phone: (401) 456-2521
Fax: (401) 456-6449
Percentage of IMGs in the program: 10%

Minimum USMLE Step 1 Score Requirement:
No limits set
Minimum USMLE Step 2 Score Requirement:
No limits set
Attempts on any step: No limits set
CS required at time of application: No
USCE Requirement: None
Cut-Off time since graduation: No limits set
Program offers couple match: Yes
Visas Sponsored or accepted: J1 visa

Texas

University of Texas Health Science Center at San Antonio Dermatology Residency Program

Specialty: Dermatology
Program name: University of Texas Health Science Center at San Antonio Program
Program code: 080-48-22-088
State: Texas
Address: University of Texas HSC San Antonio, Medicine/Dermatology MSC 7871, 7703 Floyd Curl Dr, San Antonio, TX 78229-3900
Phone: (210) 567-5673
Fax: (210) 567-4820

Percentage of IMGs in the program: 15%
Minimum USMLE Step 1 Score Requirement:
225
Minimum USMLE Step 2 Score Requirement:
225
Attempts on any step: No limits set
CS required at time of application: No
USCE Requirement: None
Cut-Off time since graduation: No limits set
Program offers couple match: Yes
Visas Sponsored or accepted: J1 visa

University of Texas at Houston Dermatology Residency Program

Specialty: Dermatology
Program name: University of Texas at Houston
Program
Program code: 080-48-21-100
State: Texas
Address: University of Texas Houston,
Department of Dermatology Suite 980,
6655 Travis St, Houston, TX 77030
Phone: (713) 500-8330
Fax: (713) 500-8321
Percentage of IMGs in the program: 8%
Minimum USMLE Step 1 Score Requirement:
230
Minimum USMLE Step 2 Score Requirement:
230

Attempts on any step: Must pass on first attempt
CS required at time of application: Yes including ECFMG certificate
USCE Requirement: None
Cut-Off time since graduation: No limits set
Program offers couple match: Yes
Visas Sponsored or accepted: J1 visa and H1b visa

University of Texas Southwestern Medical School (Austin) Dermatology Residency Program

Specialty: Dermatology
Program name: University of Texas Southwestern Medical School (Austin) Program
Program code: 080-48-12-140
NRMP Code: 2835080A1
Program type: Community-based university affiliated hospital
State: Texas
Address: University of Texas Southwestern-Austin,

Dermatology Program Suite C2 470, 601 E 15th St, Austin, TX 78701
Phone: (512) 324-7997
Fax: (512) 324-7969
Percentage of IMGs in the program: 15%

Minimum USMLE Step 1 Score Requirement: 230
Minimum USMLE Step 2 Score Requirement: 230
Attempts on any step: Must pass on first attempt
CS required at time of application: No
USCE Requirement: None
Cut-Off time since graduation: 5 years
Program offers couple match: Yes
Visas Sponsored or accepted: J1 visa

Utah

University of Utah Dermatology Residency Program

Specialty: Dermatology
Program name: University of Utah Program
Program code: 080-49-21-112
Program type: University-based
State: Utah
Address: University of Utah Medical Center, Room 4A330 SOM,
　　　30 N 1900 E, Salt Lake City, UT 84132
Phone: (801) 581-5509

Fax: (801) 581-6484
Percentage of IMGs in the program: 10%
Minimum USMLE Step 1 Score Requirement: No limits set
Minimum USMLE Step 2 Score Requirement: No limits set
Attempts on any step: No limits set
CS required at time of application: Yes including ECFMG certificate
USCE Requirement: None
Cut-Off time since graduation: No limits set
Program offers couple match: Yes
Visas Sponsored or accepted: J1 visa

Virginia

Virginia Commonwealth University Health System Dermatology Residency Program

Specialty: Dermatology
Program name: Virginia Commonwealth University Health System Program
Program code: 080-51-21-090
NRMP Code: 1743080A0
Program type: University-based
State: Virginia

Address: VCU Medical Center, PO Box 980164,
401 N 11th St, Richmond, VA 23298-0164

Phone: (804) 628-3139

Fax: (804) 827-1909

Percentage of IMGs in the program: 20%

Minimum USMLE Step 1 Score Requirement: 220

Minimum USMLE Step 2 Score Requirement: 220

Attempts on any step: No limits set

CS required at time of application: Yes including ECFMG certificate

USCE Requirement: None

Cut-Off time since graduation: No limits set

Program offers couple match: Yes

Visas Sponsored or accepted: J1 visa

Washington

University of Washington Dermatology Residency Program

Specialty: Dermatology

Program name: University of Washington Program

Program code: 080-54-31-091

NRMP Code: 1918080A0

Program type: University-based
State: Washington
Address: University of Washington School of Medicine, Box 356524 BB1353,
1959 NE Pacific St, Seattle, WA 98195-6524
Phone: (206) 685-6120
Fax: (206) 543-2489
Percentage of IMGs in the program: 10%
Minimum USMLE Step 1 Score Requirement: No limits set
Minimum USMLE Step 2 Score Requirement: No limits set
Attempts on any step: Must pass on first attempt
CS required at time of application: Yes including ECFMG certificate
USCE Requirement: None
Cut-Off time since graduation: No limits set
Program offers couple match: Yes
Visas Sponsored or accepted: J1 visa and H1b

Wisconsin

Medical College of Wisconsin Affiliated Hospitals Dermatology Residency Program

Specialty: Dermatology
Program name: Medical College of Wisconsin Affiliated Hospitals Program
Program code: 080-56-21-095
State: Wisconsin
Address: Medical College of Wisconsin, Department of Dermatology,
            9200 W Wisconsin Ave, Milwaukee, WI 53226
Phone: (414) 955-3106
Fax: (414) 955-6221
Percentage of IMGs in the program: 8%
Minimum USMLE Step 1 Score Requirement: No limits set
Minimum USMLE Step 2 Score Requirement: No limits set
Attempts on any step: No limits set
CS required at time of application: No
USCE Requirement: None
Cut-Off time since graduation: No limits set
Program offers couple match: Yes
Visas Sponsored or accepted: J1 visa

Marshfield Clinic-St Joseph's Hospital Dermatology Residency Program

Specialty: Dermatology
Program name: Marshfield Clinic-St Joseph's Hospital Program
Program code: 080-56-22-131
NRMP Code: 1780080A1
Program type: Community-based university affiliated hospital
State: Wisconsin
Address: Marshfield Clinic, Dermatology Program,
          1000 N Oak Ave, Marshfield, WI 54449
Phone: (715) 389-4151
Fax: (715) 389-4141
Percentage of IMGs in the program: 15%
Minimum USMLE Step 1 Score Requirement: 220
Minimum USMLE Step 2 Score Requirement: 220
Attempts on any step: Must pass on first attempt including CS exam
CS required at time of application: Yes including ECFMG certificate
USCE Requirement: None
Cut-Off time since graduation: 5 years
Program offers couple match: Yes
Visas Sponsored or accepted: J1 visa and H1b visa

University of Wisconsin Dermatology Residency Program

Specialty: Dermatology
Program name: University of Wisconsin Program
Program code: 080-56-21-093
NRMP Code: 1779080A0
Program type: University-based
State: Wisconsin
Address: University of Wisconsin Hospital and Clinics, Department of Dermatology,
        1 S Park St, Madison, WI 53715
Phone: (608) 287-2658
Fax: (608) 287-2676
Percentage of IMGs in the program: 20%
Minimum USMLE Step 1 Score Requirement: 220
Minimum USMLE Step 2 Score Requirement: 220
Attempts on any step: No limits set
CS required at time of application: Yes including ECFMG certificate
USCE Requirement: None
Cut-Off time since graduation: No limits set
Program offers couple match: Yes
Visas Sponsored or accepted: J1 visa

Please take 1 minute to write a review and rate our book on Amazon. We wish you a successful match. Thank you for buying our book.

If you have any questions please email us at applicantguide@yahoo.com

IMG Guide
&
Applicant Guide

www.imgguide.com
www.applicantguide.com